Dash Diet

The Comprehensive Guide To Lowering Blood Pressure
And Enhancing Health With Delectable Recipes And Meal
Plans

*(Increase Your Metabolism And Enhance Your Health
While Reducing Your Blood Pressure)*

Syed Cassidy

TABLE OF CONTENT

Chapter 1: What Is Dash Diet?

The DASH diet is a healthy eating plan devised primarily for the prevention of hypertension (high blood pressure). The diet was devised without the use of medication, but the US National Health Institute approved it. Initial studies demonstrated that a daily sodium intake of 2000 mg can reduce blood pressure. In 202 2 , American News & World Report published multiple studies on the effects of DASH on preventing diabetes, kidney failure, stroke, malignancy, and cardiovascular disease.

The Optimized DASH Diet

The first (and original) research on the DASH diet did not focus on weight loss. It was founded on the prevalent nutrition knowledge of the 2 990s. There was a need for an easy-to-follow plan based on the core basic diets because weight loss procedures did not matter to a large number of individuals at the time. This is where the DASH diet was created, and numerous research studies have been conducted since then to enhance it. In general, lowering "empty carbs" and increasing healthful fats and protein produced favorable blood pressure results. All of these enhancements are most effective when paired with a sustainable weight loss plan.

The diet emphasizes the significance of low-fat dairy products, fruits, and vegetables to the human body. Regarding the enhanced DASH diet, the latter includes a "sodium level" version. You may choose between these two DASH sodium levels that meet your daily needs:

Lower Sodium Dietary Approaches to Stop Hypertension (DASH) – You may consume 2 700 mg of sodium per day.

Standard Sodium DASH Diet – You may consume foods with a sodium content of 210 00 mg per day.

Both versions seek to reduce the amount of sodium in any diet (in which you can consume approximately 210 00 mg sodium per day). The standard sodium DASH diet is mandated by the US Dietary Association, whereas its "low-level sodium" counterpart satisfies the recommendation of 2 ,10 00 to 2 ,700 mg/day for adults aged 10 2 and older. The National Heart Association of the United States endorses 2 700 mg as the adult standard limit. (Note: if you are unsure which sodium level is appropriate for your health, consult a physician)

Not Just For Weight Reduction

The DASH diet is not only intended to promote weight loss, but it can also be used as an all-encompassing weight loss strategy. It is predicated on a daily diet of approximately 6 000 calories. Consider reducing your daily caloric intake by at least 2 ,10 00 calories if you intend to lose weight. Adjusting your regular serving objectives, regardless of your health condition, will help you choose a DASH-compatible weight loss strategy.

Reduce Sodium Intake

A key component of the DASH diet is reducing sodium (or salt) intake. Because the latter enhances flavor, fast food chains and restaurants use it as a primary constituent in their meals. Therefore, when dining in a fast food establishment or restaurant:

Choose boiled or steamed fish and request fresh herbs or lemon essence for seasoning.

Order vegetables steamed without any marinade.

Limit your consumption of condiments high in sodium. Sauces, pickles, ketchup, and mustard are examples.

Order cuisine prepared without MSG and salt.

Eliminating Unhealthy Fats

The DASH diet promotes low-cholesterol and low-saturated fat ingredients. To reduce unhealthy lipids when dining out, you should:

Choose natural culinary methods such as stir-frying, poaching, roasting, baking, broiling, grilling, and steaming.

Simple Remove any visible fat from fish, meat, and poultry. Consume a portion that is roughly the size of a deck of playing cards.

Request vinegar (or oil) as a substitute for salad dressing.

No, the DASH diet does not refer to how quickly you will consume the majority of your meals. DASH is an acronym for Dietary Approaches to Prevent Hypertension. The diet is essentially a lifetime commitment to healthy eating in order to prevent or treat hypertension or elevated blood pressure. Specifically, the diet is low in sodium – a major contributor to hypertension – and abundant in nutrient-dense foods, both of which contribute significantly to lowering high blood pressure.

If you decide to embrace and implement the DASH diet, your mission may help you reduce your blood pressure by several points in just a few weeks. And over time, as you remain steadfast in your mission, your blood pressure may drop as much as 2 8 points. Such a substantial reduction in your blood pressure significantly reduces your risk for other related health problems.

A benefit of the diet is that, as a predominantly healthful diet, it does more than just lower blood pressure. It can also help you lose weight and reduce your risk of other debilitating diseases, such as diabetes, stroke, cancer, heart attacks, and osteoporosis, among others. Now, isn't that a great offer or what?

Let's Talk About Sodium

Sodium, which is predominantly found in salt, is essential for a healthy and normally functioning body. Sodium aids in the absorption of electrolytes, which are essential for the transmission of electrical impulses in many bodily functions. Sodium enables the body to retain sufficient water and, consequently, electrolytes to function properly. Blood pressure is affected by sodium through its ability to retain water in the body. We'll discuss this further at a later time.

Also essential for deferring or preventing the onset of muscle cramps is sodium. Therefore, endurance athletes such as triathletes and ultramarathoners bring saline solutions or salt sticks to arduous competitions and training sessions.

Normal bodily function requires about 10 00 milligrams of sodium per day. Modern diets, particularly in the West, tend to provide up to 2 0 times the recommended amount. It is not surprising that hypertension is so prevalent in the world today. As previously stated, sodium primarily impacts blood pressure through water retention. How does that function?

This is how it is. The kidneys typically eliminate excess sodium from the circulation through urination. However, if the sodium level in your blood is excessively high, your kidneys may become overburdened. When this occurs, the kidney enters crisis mode and instead of flushing excess sodium through urine, it dumps it into the bloodstream.

Consider that sodium helps to retain hydration. As a result, sodium in your blood attracts water, causing your blood volume to exceed normal levels. This causes hypertension or elevated blood pressure, my friend.

There are two maximal daily sodium consumption recommendations. The Dietary Guidelines for Americans set the daily maximum at 2,6 00 milligrams, whereas the American Heart Association sets the daily maximum for adults at 2 ,10 00 milligrams. The DASH diet has two variations to accommodate the two sodium limits: standard and reduced sodium. The standard formulation permits a maximum daily consumption of 2,6 00 milligrams, which is optimal for preventing or reducing the risk of hypertension in individuals with normal blood pressure. The maximum sodium intake for those who are already hypertensive is 2 ,10 00 milligrams, which is the limit in the DASH diet version with less sodium. The standard Western (American) diet can contain as much as 8 ,000 milligrams of sodium per day. Both versions seek to reduce this amount by a substantial amount.

Let's Discuss Food

The DASH diet includes copious quantities of low-fat dairy products, fruits, grains, and vegetables, regardless of which version you choose. It also permits a certain quantity of legumes, poultry, and fish. A few times per week, small portions of fats, sweets, red meat, seeds, and almonds are also permitted. In essence, the DASH diet is a low-sodium, low-total-fat, low-saturated-fat, and low-cholesterol diet, all of which contribute significantly to hypertension.

The DASH diet is also one in which daily caloric intake is limited to a certain range, specifically between 2 ,10 00 and

2,000 calories. As a result, consuming the appropriate quantities or portions is essential for successfully managing hypertension with a diet. To give you an idea of which foods are ideal and how much you should consume daily, here is a list of the diet's recommended foods and daily portions:

Vegetables

Greens, sweet potatoes, broccoli, carrots, and tomatoes are among the most beneficial vegetables for the DASH diet. They are rich in dietary fiber, vitamins, and essential minerals such as potassium and magnesium. You can consume four to five servings per day, with each serving consisting of a cup of raw green leafy vegetables or a half cup of cooked or uncooked cut vegetables.

When purchasing frozen or canned vegetables, examine the label carefully. Stick to items that are labeled "low sodium" or "no salt added" and similar phrases.

Complete Grains

This dietary group may contain whole-wheat pasta, whole-wheat rice, cereal, and whole-wheat bread. Ensure that the labels read "Made from 2 00% Whole Wheat" or "2 00% Whole Grain" or something similar. You may consume up to eight portions per day. A serving consists of one slice of whole-wheat bread, half a cup of prepared pasta, rice, or cereal, and one ounce of dry cereal.

Regarding the DASH diet, I strongly suggest consuming more whole grains than anything else. First, it is more satisfying and will stave off appetite longer. Moreover, whole grains contain substantially more nutrients and dietary fiber than their refined counterparts.

Dairy foods such as cheese, yogurt, and milk are excellent sources of protein, vitamin D, and calcium; however, if you make poor choices, you may consume an excessive amount of saturated fat, which is discouraged by the DASH diet. So, how do you proceed? Simple, opt for the fat-free or low-fat alternatives. You may consume up to three servings per day, with one serving consisting of a cup of 2 % or skim milk, 2 .10 ounces of partially skimmed cheese, and one cup of low-fat yogurt. You can add a serving of your preferred fruit for a healthier and tastier twist. And regarding...

Fruits

Fruits are rich in magnesium, potassium, and dietary fiber while being extremely low in cholesterol, with the exception of coconuts. They are excellent as a nibble or garnish for your DASH main dishes. You may consume up to five servings per day, with a serving consisting of one-half cup (canned, frozen, or raw), one medium-sized fruit, or four ounces of natural fruit juice (not juice drinks). If you choose canned varieties, check the label to ensure that no added sugar has been included.

Just use caution when consuming citrus fruits and their liquids. They have the potential to alter the efficacy of certain types of medications. If you are currently taking medication and would like to include citrus fruits like grapefruit in your diet, you should verify with your doctor first.

Legumes, Seeds, And Nuts

These foods are superb sources of protein, potassium, and magnesium: lentils, peas, kidney beans, sunflower seeds, and almonds. However, there is more! Legumes, seeds, and nuts are also loaded with dietary fiber and phytochemicals, the latter of which is extremely beneficial for lowering the risk of heart disease and certain types of cancer. You may consume up to five servings of these goods per week. Please note that this is weekly and not daily. The reason for the weekly restriction is that they are extremely calorie dense, or very high in calories. This dish contains 2 tablespoons of seeds, 2 /6 cup of nuts, and 1 cup of cooked peas or legumes per serving.

Although nuts are high in calories, especially from fat, the fats they contain are healthful or beneficial: omega-6 fatty acids and monounsaturated fats. Remember to consume them in moderation because, as stated previously, they are extremely high in calories.

Fish, Poultry, And Lean Meats Are Good Sources Of Protein

Lean portions of red meat are an excellent source of zinc, iron, B vitamins, and protein; however, the DASH diet limits daily consumption to a maximum of 6 ounces. When consuming poultry, focus on the breast, which contains the least amount of fat, and eliminate the fat and skin prior to cooking. Instead of frying, try roasting, grilling, broiling, or baking, which are all healthier and reduce dietary cholesterol. Tuna, herring, and salmon are examples of fish that contain heart-healthy lipids (omega-6 fatty acids) that can assist in lowering cholesterol levels. You may consume up to six daily servings of fish, lean meat, and poultry.

Sweets

The DASH diet is incredibly nutritious and not lethal. Don't be surprised if you can satiate your sweet tooth while following the DASH diet to lower your blood pressure. However, moderation is the key to success here. You are permitted no more than five servings of sweets per week on the regimen. Indeed, weekly rather than daily. A standard serving would consist of one cup of lemonade, one-half cup of sorbet, and one tablespoon of marmalade, jelly, or sugar.

Choose low- or non-fat sweets, such as low-fat pastries, graham crackers, hard candies, jelly beans, fruit ices, and sorbet, when satisfying your sweet tooth.

To satiate your cravings, you may be tempted to consume more products that contain sugar substitutes such as sucralose, aspartame, or stevia. This may get you off the hook, but it does not help you control your cravings or sweet appetite. The next time you have a craving and there is no sugar-free option available, there is a good chance that you will cave because you never had the opportunity to strengthen your willpower. You should choose healthier alternatives such as low-fat or non-fat milk. Better yet, learn to consume more water.

Oils And Dietary Fats

Even on the DASH diet, it is unwise to wholly eliminate fat from your diet. Why? This is due to the fact that dietary fat serves two very important functions: it allows your body to assimilate and utilize several essential vitamins, and it strengthens your immune system. The question here is whether or not you are going too far. Certainly, too much of a good thing – particularly dietary fat – can be bad, as it significantly increases the likelihood that you will develop obesity, diabetes, or a heart condition in the future.

The DASH diet takes into account the need for and moderation of dietary fat consumption, and as a result, it allows you to consume less than 6 0 percent of your daily caloric needs from it. In addition, the diet stresses the importance of selecting healthy lipids, specifically monounsaturated fats.

Under the diet, you may consume up to three servings per day, with one serving including, among other things, two tablespoons of your preferred salad dressing, one tablespoon of mayonnaise, one teaspoon of virgin coconut oil, and one teaspoon of soft margarine. Avoid unhealthy fats, such as saturated and trans fats, which are typically present in highly processed foods such as French fries, baked products, and crackers. Becoming accustomed to reading product labels will be of great benefit.

Caffeine And Alcohol

Caffeine and alcohol can also increase blood pressure, in addition to sodium. Although the DASH diet does not address caffeine consumption because a direct correlation between caffeine consumption and hypertension (chronic high blood pressure) has not yet been established, it is a well-known fact that caffeine can cause temporary increases in blood pressure. Therefore, if you already have hypertension or believe that consuming caffeinated beverages raises your blood pressure, it is best to avoid them altogether. safer is better than sorry. Or, if you absolutely must have your coffee dose, opt for the decaffeinated version.

Additionally, excessive alcohol consumption can result in elevated blood pressure. In light of this, the Dietary Guidelines for Americans restrict alcohol consumption to no more than two drinks per day for men and one drink per day for women. However, given that alcohol provides no tangible health benefits, the hypertension risk associated with it is not worthwhile. If you truly want to manage your hypertension or reduce your risks for it, you should discard the item.

Weight Loss

As previously mentioned, weight loss is a desirable prospective side effect of the DASH diet, despite not being its primary purpose. The reason for weight loss under the program is straightforward: healthy diet. Healthy eating encompasses both the quality and quantity of food.

If you consume more than 2,000 calories per day on a daily basis, it is likely that you will lose weight on the regimen. This is because an average daily caloric intake of 2,000 calories will result in a caloric deficit for you, i.e., you will expend more calories than you consume.

Chapter 2: What To Consume And What To Avoid

One of the benefits of the DASH diet is that it includes a wide variety of foods, providing you with numerous options. Moreover, it is straightforward.

DASH Friendly Foods

The DASH diet permits the consumption of seven dietary groups:

On the DASH diet, it is recommended to consume four to five servings of vegetables daily. Magnesium, vitamins, potassium, and fiber are all abundant in vegetables. Limit your sodium intake, but pay close attention to the nutritional content. Beans are a healthy option, but if you choose canned beans, examine the nutrition label for sodium content. The vitamin A and fiber content of sweet potatoes enhances the functionality of blood vessels. Winter squash, cauliflower, broccoli, spinach, carrots, kale, beetroot, garlic, onions, and tomatoes are additional options.

Fruits – Just as with vegetables, you should consume at least four to five servings of fruit each day for the fiber and vital energy they provide, which promote correct body function. Fruits are available in dried, frozen, canned, and raw forms. Make sure you have read the nutritional label on tinned fruits to determine if they contain added sugar. The majority of fruits are rich in magnesium, fiber, and potassium, and low in cholesterol. Apples, bananas, pears, peaches, dates, grapes, mangoes, nectarines, strawberries, blueberries, raspberries, raisins, pineapples, oranges, and melons are examples of common fruits permitted on the DASH diet.

Whole Grains – To increase your nutrient and fiber intake, consume seven to eight servings of whole grains each day. You can contemplate various cereals. Avoid adorning your pasta and bread with cheese, cream, or butter. Consider whole-wheat pasta, brown rice, popcorn, whole oats, quinoa, and whole-wheat bread, among other healthful options.

Consider both low-fat and fat-free dairy products when deciding which dairy products to incorporate into your diet. These are rich in vitamin D, calcium, and protein. This can be a cup of yogurt, milk, or cheese weighing 2 .10 ounces. Other alternatives include low-fat, skim, and fat-free milk, low-fat and fat-free cheese, and low-fat and fat-free yogurt. Because coconut and almond milk lack dairy properties, they cannot replace dairy products. Potassium, calcium, and vitamin D are essential for the absorption of nutrients found in milk.

Lean Protein – The DASH diet requires that you consume at least six servings of poultry, lean meat, or fish per day. Lean and skinless meat are excellent sources of protein, zinc, iron, and vitamin B complex. Seafood and fish, which provide Omega 6 and help lower cholesterol, are among the options you can consider. To limit salt and preservative intake, however, you should prioritize fresh food over tinned. You may broil, grill, or roast, but you should avoid frying. Also available are fresh eggs, with one fresh egg equaling one serving, and lean poultry (always ensure the skin is removed).

Nuts (Legumes and Seeds) - Include five to six servings of beans, legumes, nuts, and seeds in your weekly meal plan. Magnesium, phytochemicals, protein, and fiber are abundant in these foods. As the majority of these items are high in calories, you should be mindful of your intake. A single ration of nuts is two tablespoons. This group of nutrients includes, among others, pistachios, lentils, kidney beans, peas, cashews, peanuts, and almonds.

According to nutritionists, you should consume two to three servings of lipids and oils per day. These are essential for immune system health and nutrient absorption. Even then, you must exercise caution and control the amount you use because excessive lipids and oils can lead to obesity, diabetes, and cardiovascular disease if left unchecked. One serving can consist of one teaspoon of mayonnaise, one tablespoon of salad dressing, light margarine, or one tablespoon of vegetable oil. Also available are coconut oil, extra virgin olive oil, and groundnut oil.

Sugars and treats – Surprise! The DASH diet permits you to consume no more than five servings of sugar per week. This plan does not entirely prohibit sweets. However, you should strive for those that contain less fat. Jelly beans, low-fat granola biscuits or bars, and fruit ice are ideal examples of foods that comprise a serving. Sugar, natural honey, agave syrup, and maple syrup are a few of the sweeteners you can consider. The majority of these are natural sweeteners, making them an excellent option.

Foods That Are Limited

DASH restricts the consumption of artificial sweeteners, salted nuts, red meat, sweets and added sugars, saturated and Trans-fats, high-fat snacks, high-sodium salad dressing, dairy with high-fat or full-cream milk, high-sodium foods, caffeine, and cigarettes. You should also moderate your alcohol consumption. Therefore, if you have issues with alcohol, you should seek assistance, as it can be difficult to reduce consumption.

DASH Foods for Vegetarians and Vegans

The DASH diet is not restricted to lean individuals. Vegetarians and vegans can appreciate the DASH diet by substituting plant-based proteins for animal proteins. Proteins cannot be eliminated from your diet because your body does not store them. The amino acids prevalent in these two sources of protein are dissimilar. Animal proteins contain a greater variety of amino acids than plant proteins. In addition, the majority of plant proteins lack essential amino acids such as lysine, isoleucine, methionine, and tryptophan. In comparison to meat, legumes are the greatest source of plant-based protein. Consequently, you should consume at least three servings of peanuts, tofu, beans, and peas.

You must be aware that vegan requirements for the DASH diet are quite distinct. You must replace dairy products with soy products such as soy beverages, soy yogurt, and sour cream. All soy-based products are acceptable. Additionally, you must locate substitutes for poultry, fish, and lean meats among wheat meat, tempeh, and tofu.

In terms of legumes, seeds, and almonds, you have unique options for meeting your potassium and protein needs. However, you must exercise portion control with care. You can also consider amaranth and quinoa, which are high-protein nutrients.

Planning Your DASH Diet

Your DASH diet success begins with the food you purchase. Before you go retail shopping, you'll need to:

Make an inventory. You must first determine the meals you will eat during the week, create a list of the necessary ingredients, and then go grocery shopping with this list in order to avoid the temptation to purchase unhealthy food.

Consume food first. Avoid grocery purchasing when you're hungry, as everything will seem appealing. It can be difficult to resist the temptation to purchase foods high in sodium and cholesterol.

Resist the allure of displays and sales when you go shopping. Consider purchasing fresh food because processed foods typically contain high levels of sodium. Additionally, you must shop on the store's sides because this is where the fresh produce is located. In particular, stock up on fruits, low-fat dairy products, vegetables, nuts, cereals, seeds and legumes, as well as lean meats, fish, and poultry, as well as condiments, seasonings, and spreads. Lastly, be sure to examine the labels of packaged foods to determine whether or not they are suitable for your diet.

DASH-Compatible Cooking Methods

Cookware and kitchen appliances can make it simpler to adhere to the DASH diet. Nonstick cookware, a vegetable steamer, an oven, and a spice mill or garlic press are some of the useful items that you need. You should also strive for culinary methods that minimize the use of fat and sodium. Start

Chapter 3: How Does Dash Diet Works

You may be familiar with the DASH Diet for Hypertension. Well, it is currently one of the most popular diet rlan available, and it may be more than a fad. This diet program was created by the US Department of Health and Human Services' National Institutes of Health and is based on nutritional facts.

DASH is an abbreviation of Dietaru This baisallu refers to Stor Hurertenion and provides information on how to reduce your blood pressure through diet. The premise of the diet plan is to instruct men and women with hypertension and high blood pressure on how to consume more healthily and reduce their blood pressure and the risk of associated diseases. High blood pressure is often a problem that can be avoided by leading a healthy lifestyle; however, once a person has high blood pressure, it can only be managed.

Having high blood pressure is a serious matter that can lead to diseases such as coronary artery disease, dementia, stroke, and ultimately heart failure. Up to 6 6 percent of men and women currently have hypertension or elevated blood pressure. That's one-third of the adult population, so there's a high likelihood that you or someone you know will be diagnosed with the disease.

By adhering to a few guidelines, the DASH Diet for Hypertension can assist you in lowering your blood pressure as well as your risk for a number of related conditions. For example, one of the primary recommendations of the weight loss program is to reduce your sodium intake to between 2,6 00 and 2 ,10 00 mg per day. This may give the impression that you are still receiving a substantial amount of odium, but in reality it is not very much. Consider some of the items you may ingest on a daily basis.

Did you know that a quarter rounder with cheese contains about 2 ,2 90 milligrams of sodium? If you restrict yourself to 2 ,10 00 milligrams per day, that is your entire daily allowance. Even at 2,6 00 per day, there are still over 10 0 instances of the suggested daily error. Even if you believe you will suffer from a health problem and become sad, you should be cautious. Historically, condiments and dressings have been notorious for their high sodium content.

So, what will you ultimately consume on The DASH Diet?

Plenty of vegetables and fruits per day rather than sweets and desserts.

Dietary fiber-rich foods are an alternative to refined carbohydrates.

Low-fat and fat-free milk products instead of whole milk products.

Water and slub oda were added to ugaru oft beverages.

The DASH Diet is not just a dietary plan; it also recommends some healthy lifestyle changes.

Start a workout regimen whether or not your blood pressure is normal.

Tru must get at least thirty minutes of daily rhuisal exercise.

Determine your own weight reduction objectives.

If you take resrirtion medication for high blood pressure, remember to take it every day.

With such conventional ene advice, it's not surprising. The DASH Diet is gaining such popularity at the present. This is a diet that makes logic and has the potential to help you lose weight and maintain your health. Even persons with healthy blood pressure can typically benefit from the DASH Diet and adopting a high-fiber, low-fat, low-sodium diet.

This diet will not only enable you to "hed round," but it will also help save your life.

How Does 6 Phase Liver Detox Diet Cleansing Work?

You must have learned about the cirrhosis of the liver in biology class. Your liver is the largest internal organ in your body and performs more than 10 00 different functions. One of the most important functions of the liver is that it filters out toxins and substances that enter the body and prevents them from entering the bloodstream. Your liver becomes lethargic over time due to accumulated toxins. It is crucial to eliminate the toxic accumulation in the liver, which is why a liver detox is crucial. One of the most effective methods of liver detoxification is the liver detox diet.

Preparing It

Before beginning a liver detox diet, you must meticulously plan everything out. Planning is essential since you must prepare your body for the diet. Preparing the bodu will maximize the efficacy of the detox program. Now the question is how you will prepare. The first thing you must do is abstain from caffeine, alcohol, unhealthy food, sugar, and meat. Before beginning the detox diet, consume only vegetables and fruits for one week. Reduce your sugar intake and increase your consumption of fluids and whole wheat bread. Continue the detox diet in three phases over the course of one week.

First Phase

The initial phase of the detox diet will last between the first and third day. You must survive the olelu on liuid. Take 2 0 to 2 2 glasses of water with a dash of fresh lemon juice. This will aid in detoxification and eliminate accumulated waste. Stau is distinguished from other beverages and dairy products. This will calm your digestive system and liver. You may experience some fatigue; have no fear. This occurs because all the water is being flushed out of your septic system. During this period, you may drink roemaru tea if you so choose.

Second step

For the next three days, the third phase of the liver detoxification regimen will continue. You san inslude fruits, vegetables and semi solid food in your diet during this phase. The designation for organically cultivated fruits and vegetables. You must continue to consume 2 2 glasses of water during this phase. Fresh fruit juices are excellent for liver detox. Therefore, each morning consists of orange, apple, celery, or carrot juice. Every night, consume a vegetable bouillon consisting of sarrot, rinash rotato, and broccoli. You may continue drinking roemaru tea even in this course.

Third Period

The third phase of the liver cleansing diet will only last for seven days. Include in your diet 2 2 glasses of water, green tea, fresh produce, and organically grown vegetables. Raw vegetables are good for liver detoxifisation. Nevertheless, you may "team your vegetable" if you so choose. To discontinue the diet program, return to your normal diet gradually. Stay away from alcohol for at least one week after the end of the diet program.

Chapter 4: Benefits Of The Dash Diet

In order to lower blood pressure, the DASH diet recommends low sodium intake. A diet low in sodium reduces the likelihood of developing elevated blood pressure and becoming hypertensive.

Following the DASH diet can help those who are already hypertensive reduce the effects of the disease. The DASH diet endorses the recommendation that hypertensive patients consume low-sodium foods.

The dash diet can aid in weight loss. This is due to the fact that the DASH diet includes foods that are minimal in fat or, better yet, fat free. This indicates that you will consume lipids that are not harmful to your health.

The DASH diet also encourages fruit and vegetable consumption. Fruits and vegetables are essential mineral and vitamin sources. Additionally, it aids in the elimination of saturated lipids and cholesterol from the diet. Cholesterol and saturated lipids are the primary causes of hypertension.

Identify Unproductive Behaviors

Self-reflection will be a part of taking steps toward healthier food, but this does not require a complete life overhaul. Ask yourself what you are generally pleased with about your current food habits and what you would like to change. This type of reflection is frequently extraordinarily beneficial because it prompts you to consider your goals and actions. You are the lord of yourself, and the information you generate about yourself is roughly equivalent to the information an expert can provide.

Keep in mind that this activity does not originate from a place of pessimism or self-analysis, but rather from a place of legitimate self-reflection. You should be delighted with the positive steps you are taking to improve your health while also monitoring the behaviors that may be preventing you from achieving your goals. The week-to-week habit tracker that accompanies your 28-day plan will be an incredibly helpful tool for facilitating self-reflection and putting you on the path to improved habits.

However, what is a pointless disposition? It is neither negative nor harmful, but it may be futile. Despite the fact that everyone leads a unique existence, there are a number of common tendencies within this category that frequently emerge among my private practice clients.

Frequent suppers out: There is nothing negative about eating out; however, when we dine out frequently, our intake of calories and sodium is exceptionally high, making it difficult to manage weight and lower blood pressure.

Lack of planning snacks: The time between lunch and dinner can be deceiving for some people. When hunger is unchecked during this period, it frequently leads to either consuming whatever is nearby or being so ravenous at dinnertime that poor decisions are frequently made.

Overusing oil: Oil is a healthy source of dietary fat and a method for enhancing the flavor of meals; however, using more than 2 tablespoon of oil at a time is an easy way to overconsume calories that do not provide much satiety in return.

Consuming due to stress or fatigue: Call a friend, go for a walk, cleanse up, read a book, and exercise. There are a variety of alternatives to food that can assist you in avoiding the common pitfall of using food to deal with your emotions. Find the one that works best for you, and remember that there is never a bad time for a healthy snack such as a piece of fruit.

Setting Aims

Success in losing weight and lowering heart rate depends largely on your ability to adhere to the DASH diet plan. You should establish goals that are narrowly focused on this. When you have successfully adopted the healthy, modified DASH eating style, only then will your health and weight alter. Regarding vegetable consumption, for instance, we should investigate how to formulate a SMART objective:

Specific: Be quite certain. For instance, I will increase my weekly vegetable consumption.

Measurable: Assign a number to it. For example, I consume five servings of vegetables per day.

Achievable: Evaluate your current situation relative to where you should be. If you are currently consuming zero servings per day, it would be unreasonable to increase to five.

Significant: Eating more vegetables is directly relevant to your ultimate goal of adhering to the DASH diet and plays a tremendous role in lowering your pulse and keeping you full, nourished, and satiated.

Time Limited: Setting a deadline holds you accountable for your objective. You should consider your 28-day program period as a reasonable starting point for establishing goals. Alternatively, you should divide objectives into one-week increments.

Let me begin by recommending a medium- to long-term perspective to those who may be considering reasonable weight loss objectives.

Thinking in terms of months rather than years will help you appreciate excellent dieting consistently and eliminate the unreasonable expectations that some individuals place on themselves when attempting to become more physically fit. We know, from a health perspective, that a modest weight loss of 10 to 2 0 percent of one's current weight is all that is required to further develop metabolic functioning. In my private practice, I observe that once my clients have lost approximately this amount of weight, they frequently report better performance at work, their abdominal outline diminishes, their garments begin fitting better, and they no longer feel the same desire to pursue additional weight loss.

To put this in perspective, a weight loss of 10 to 2 0 percent for a 200-pound individual equates to between 2 0 and 20 pounds. This is not a small number, but it is by no means exorbitant in the grand scheme of things. Those wishing to lose weight should see between four ounces and one pound of weight loss per week as an indication of progress.

Please keep in mind that the rate of calamity will vary from person to person. Getting in shape is difficult, and your success on this program is not determined by your weight loss. Your capacity to begin and maintain weight loss will depend on a number of factors, most notably your capacity to adhere to a diet and exercise plan within this program that you can enjoy and support over the long haul. In the initial DASH diet studies, participants reduced their heart rate and improved their health without experiencing weight loss. Regardless of your goal, the DASH diet will result in a healthier you.

Chapter 5: The Dash Diet: Healthy Eating To Lower Blood Pressure

Wait for Dietaru Arroashe to arrive at Stor Hurertenon. The DASH diet is a healthful eating regimen designed to treat or prevent hypertension. The DASH diet incorporates foods rich in potassium, calcium, and magnesium. These nutrients help regulate blood pressure. Dietary foods that are high in sugar, saturated fat, and added sugar. The DASH diet has been shown to reduce blood pressure in as little as two weeks. The diet can also reduce blood levels of low-density lipoprotein (LDL or "bad") cholesterol. High blood pressure and high LDL cholesterol levels are two of the most significant risk factors for heart disease and stroke.

DASH DIET AND SODIUM

The DASH diet contains less sodium than a typical American diet, which may contain 6 ,8 00 milligrams (mg) or more per day. The standard DASH diet limits sodium to 2,6 00 mg a dau. It satisfies the Dietary Guidelines' recommendation for Americans to limit their daily sodium intake to less than 2,6 00 mg. This is approximately the amount of sugar in one teaspoon of table salt. A lower dose version of DASH restricts the dosage to 2 ,10 00 mg per day. You must select the variant of the diet that meets your nutritional requirements. Consult with your doctor if you are unsure of the ideal sodium level for you.

DASH DIET: WHAT TO EAT

The DASH diet is a flexible and well-balanced dietary plan that helps maintain a heart-healthy diet for life. It is simple to adhere to a diet consisting of food from our grocery store. The DASH diet emphasizes fruits, vegetables, and whole grains. It includes fat-free or low-fat dairy, meat, grains, beans, and nuts. It restricts foods high in saturated fat, such as fatty meats and full-fat dairy products. When following the DASH diet, it is essential to choose foods that are:

Rsh on rotaium, sodium, magnesium, iron, and rotenium.

Low in saturated fat Low in cholesterol

WHAT EXACTLY IS THE DASH DIET?

The Dash Diet is not strictly a diet, but rather a diet designed for individuals with hypertension. High blood pressure can result in strokes, cardiac failure, heart attack, and even blindness, so a healthy diet is necessary for survival.

Diet plays a significant influence in hypertension. However, many patients are overconfident in blood-pressure-lowering medications. Instead of focusing on the appropriate diet, individuals focus on the incorrect diet, resulting in the need for medication and surgery.

The DASH Diet can assist in reducing blood pressure. In addition, many nutritionists consider the Dash Diet to be one of the healthiest eating plans.

The lower your blood pressure, the less sodium you consume.

With the Dash Diet, you will consume more fruits and vegetables, low-fat dairy products, legumes, and seeds.

fewer fatty meats, whole milk products, sugary beverages, candies, and sodium chloride.

You can also consume the Dash Diet to lose weight. When individuals adhere to the Dash Diet and increase their physical activity, they lose weight and enhance metabolic properties, such as insulin sensitivity. However, when compared to low-carb regimens, the DASH diet alone is not as effective a weight loss strategy. The Dash Diet emphasizes health improvement. When the DASH diet is combined with exercise and calorie restriction, blood pressure can be reduced even further.

This book concludes with recipes that will help you lose weight and decrease your blood pressure.

The acronym for the DASH diet is "Dietary Approaches to Stop Hypertension." The Dash Diet is intended for a specific group of individuals with high blood pressure. Nonetheless, this regimen has been shown to aid in weight loss.

Individuals following the DASH diet are encouraged to consume an abundance of fruits and vegetables. Additionally, you are advised to consume whole grains, lean meats, and some healthful fats. Since its inception, the DASH diet has been modified to permit weight loss and blood pressure reduction simultaneously.

A diet abundant in protein, fiber, potassium, magnesium, and calcium (fruits and vegetables, beans, nuts, whole grains, and low-fat dairy products) has repeatedly been shown to reduce high blood pressure.

Recent research has demonstrated that the Dash Diet can also help reduce inflammatory markers, lower the risk of kidney disease (a common complication of hypertension), and lower lipoprotein levels.

While a doctor's typical recommendation for lowering blood pressure is to reduce sodium intake, the DASH diet demonstrates that lowering blood pressure through diet is the result of integrating several nutrients. The difference lies in the synergy between DASH nutrients. The DASH diet has been shown to reduce blood pressure in a variety of populations.

HYPERTENSION

Blood pressure is the measurement of the force of blood flow within the blood vessels. Only half of the nearly 210 million Germans with elevated blood pressure have it under control. Approximately 7 million adults with elevated blood pressure are unaware of their condition and do nothing to treat it. One of the many causes of high blood pressure is an unhealthy diet.

Damaged arteries, aneurysms, an enlarged heart, transient ischemic attacks, stroke, dementia, kidney failure, retinopathy, sexual dysfunction in men, sleep apnea, and bone loss are among the negative side effects. Controlling blood pressure is therefore essential for disease prevention.

Blood pressure is measured in "millimeters of mercury" (mmHG). Two measurements are made. The first value represents the pressure in the blood vessels when the heart muscle contracts, while the second value measures the pressure when the heart muscle relaxes. A blood pressure reading greater than 2 8 0/90 mmHg is considered high. Between 2 20/80 mmHg and 2 6 9/89 mmHg is the preload. Prehypertension will likely result in hypertension. In addition, changes in lifestyle and diet will induce high blood pressure. Several nutrients found in abundance on the DASH diet are known to play an essential role in regulating blood pressure.

WHAT IS THE FASTEST AND MOST SAFE WAY TO REDUCE BLOOD PRESSURE?

Your diet has a significant impact on your blood pressure, and eating healthier foods can help control and even rectify high blood pressure. The DASH Diet is intended to help you maintain a healthy heart and avoid consuming foods that raise blood pressure. Maintaining a healthy heart requires an understanding of healthy eating practices.

The mere notion of a doctor's appointment can elevate the blood pressure of many individuals. Visiting the doctor can be nerve-wracking, particularly if you are unsure of your health status. You may be pondering if there is a quick way to lower your blood pressure to prevent hypertension.

Why do you have elevated blood pressure?

It is normal for blood pressure to momentarily increase during physical activity or after consuming a cup of coffee. However, if your heart is continuously pumping more blood than usual or if your blood vessels become stiffer, your blood pressure can remain elevated over time. Eventually, this will result in elevated blood pressure.

Another factor is an excessively salty diet. Additionally, obesity contributes to elevated blood pressure. Certain medications can induce hypertension as a side effect.

You may be aware that a blood pressure reading contains two numbers (for example, the optimal blood pressure is 2 20/80 or lower). Blood pressure is considered "normal" up to 2 29/88 .

Why is it hazardous to rapidly reduce blood pressure?

Before we delve into specific instances, let's examine why it is hazardous to rapidly lower blood pressure. Your heart and blood vessels transport blood to all regions of your body, including large, life-sustaining organs.

The example is your lungs and especially your brain. Large drops in blood pressure can abruptly deprive the brain of the blood and oxygen it requires. This can result in a stroke and irreversible cerebral damage.

What can I do about my critically high blood pressure?

High blood pressure, also known as the "silent killer," typically has few symptoms. Occasionally, however, a patient may be requested to monitor their blood pressure. Numerous symptoms exist, including headache, chest discomfort, shortness of breath, nausea, and loss of balance. These symptoms may indicate critically high blood pressure, also known as a hypertensive crisis, if your first and second blood pressure readings are greater than 2 80 and 2 20 respectively.

In this situation, DO NOT attempt to reduce your blood pressure on your own. A hypertensive crisis is a potentially fatal emergency situation.

Does sodium have an impact on my blood pressure?

Yes! If you consume an excessive amount of sodium, the extra water stored in your body can increase your blood pressure.

Our daily salt requirements are met by the sodium already present in our prepared foods, such as bread, breakfast cereals, and ready-to-eat meals, making it simple to control the salt content of your diet. This leaves no room for adding salt while preparing or dining.

Read food labels to identify foods that are high in sodium. You should consume less than 2,6 00 milligrams of sodium per day (and preferably more than 2 ,10 00 mg).

Is Fish Beneficial To Blood Pressure?

The consumption of fish with a high concentration of omega-6 fatty acids reduces blood pressure in many individuals. Salmon and mackerel are rich in omega-6 minerals and should be included in a diet that promotes cardiac health. Be wary of mercury-containing fish like swordfish, halibut, and tuna. It is highly recommended to avoid these species of fish.

Does Yoga Reduce Blood Pressure?

Numerous factors, including B. sedentary lifestyle, inadequate diet, obesity, smoking, stress, and family history, can contribute to high blood pressure.

Eating a nutritious diet and engaging in regular exercise can help you manage your blood pressure. Yoga is another natural and secure method for controlling high blood pressure. Yoga is an ancient method for staying fit and resolving numerous health issues. Yoga's health benefits are extremely popular.

Yoga exercises involve a specific breathing pattern that can reduce blood pressure and tension. Yoga will also enhance your heart's functionality. Yoga has a beneficial effect on the body and psyche and is an effective method for reducing blood pressure.

Orzo and vegetables in a barbecue sauce with peppery prawns. Ingredient Checklist

• 2 cup whole-grain orzo;

• 6 scallions;

• 4 tablespoons olive oil, divided;

• 4 cups coarsely chopped zucchini;

• 2 cup coarsely chopped bell pepper;

• Lemon wedges to put on the table

• 2 pound peeled and deveined jumbo shrimp, thawed if frozen (see Tip);

• 2 teaspoon paprika;

• 1 teaspoon garlic powder;

• 1 teaspoon crushed dried oregano;

• 1/2 teaspoon ground pepper;

• 1/7 teaspoon cayenne pepper;

List of things to do

1. Put the shrimp in a medium-sized bowl. In a small bowl, mix together the paprika, garlic powder, oregano, pepper, and cayenne.
2. Sprinkle the spice mix over the shrimp, toss to coat, and set aside.
3. Bring a lot of water to a boil in a large pot. Easy cook orzo according to the directions on the package, then drain.
4. Put it back in the hot pot, cover it, and keep it warm.
5. Slice the scallions, making sure to separate the white and green parts.
6. In a medium-sized pan, heat 2 tablespoon of oil over medium-high heat.
7. Add the white parts of the scallions, zucchini, bell pepper, and celery.

8. Cook, stirring every so often, for about 10 minutes, or until the vegetables are crisp-tender.
9. Add the tomatoes and easy cook for another 5-10 minutes, until they are soft.
10. Mix the vegetables in with the orzo in the pot.
11. Add salt and mix together.
12. Heat the last tablespoon of oil in the same pan over medium heat.
13. Add the shrimp and easy cook for 5-10 minutes, turning them once, until they are opaque.
14. Put barbecue sauce on top.
15. About a minute of cooking and stirring is all it takes to coat the shrimp.
16. Mix the vegetables and serve them with the shrimp.
17. If you want, you can serve it with wedges of lemon on top.

Cooked With Quinoa, Brussels Sprouts, And Broccoli Is Halibut.

List of Ingredients

- Butter, unsalted, 4 tablespoons, warmed

- 4 cups of quinoa cooked Sun-dried tomato chunks, about 2 8 cup

- Kalamata olives, chopped, 2 8 cup

- Parsley or Fennel Fronds 4 Tablespoons of chopped fresh Italian parsley

- 2 pound trimmed and sliced Brussels sprouts

- 2 trimmed and sliced fennel bulb

- 2 -teaspoon and 2 -teaspoon of olive oil

- 20 teaspoons of salt, split

- 20 tsp. finely ground pepper

- halibut fillet, split into four 2 -pound servings

- 8 minced and split garlic cloves

- a squeeze of fresh lemon juice, about a third cup

Soup Made With Lentils And Sage

1 cup heavy cream or sub for soy cream
8 cloves garlic, minced
4 tbs lemon juice
2 tbs butter

2 lb Cannellini beans (dry)
2 yellow onion, chopped
10 cups vegetable broth
10 fresh sage leaves

Directions:

1. Soak beans overnight to soften them, then strain and set aside before cooking.
2. In a large saucepan, cook onion and garlic in butter over medium heat.
3. Cook Simple Cook the onion for 2 minutes before adding the sage, lemon juice, stirring, and cooking on

low heat for an additional 5-10 minutes.

4. Add the broth, then bring to a simmer.

5. Add in legumes, then cover. Check the soup frequently and add water as necessary.

6. Cook Easy Simmer the soup mixture for 5-10 minutes, then test the beans for doneness.

7. Remove Simple Once simmering, remove the broth from the heat and allow it to cool.

8. Once soup is warm but not boiling,

9. blend it in large quantities until smooth. Return the broth to the saucepan and stir in the cream.

10. Stir thoroughly before heating to temperature.

11. If preferred, garnish the soup with fresh sage before serving.

Chapter 6: Fish, Poultry, Dry Beans, And Nuts Comprise Food Pyramid Tier 8 B.

The next stratum of the Dash diet pyramid includes meat, poultry, fish, dry beans, fresh eggs, and nuts. This food group provides the body with protein, iron, zinc, and some vitamin B; consequently, consuming foods from this group keeps the body healthy and robust. Select leaner cuts of meat whenever possible, and always simple Remove the skin from chicken, turkey, and other poultry.

The benefits of ingesting foods within this category

Fresh eggs are classified with meats because they are an exceptional source of iron and protein. When deciding how many fresh eggs to consume in one sitting, it is important to remember that the majority of the fresh egg's fat is located in the yolk.

Beans contain a significant quantity of fiber. They are a low-fat, protein-rich food source. In addition to being an excellent source of iron and protein, nuts also contain a high proportion of healthful fats.

Tier 10 - Fats, Oils, Sweets, Supplements

The level of the dietary pyramid that includes fats, oils, sweets, and supplements is the apex. Each component of this food group should be consumed in no more than moderate quantities. Calcium, vitamin D, vitamin B2 2, and supplements make up the second group.

Because many individuals do not consume enough of these vitamins and because our bodies produce less of them as we age, the Dash diet pyramid suggests incorporating calcium, vitamin D, and vitamin B2 2 into your daily routine. This is because the loss of these vitamins as we age emphasizes the importance of supplementation with these particular nutrients.

Make informed choices regarding the oils and lipids you consume.

When selecting lipids and oils, you should exercise care and deliberation. Omega-6 and omega-6 fatty acids are not naturally produced by the human organism. Consequently, we call certain fatty acids "essential." The only method to obtain them in any quantity is to consume foods. These lipids protect against cardiovascular disease and reduce inflammation within the body. The majority of these lipids are found in foods such as fish, nuts, and specific types of vegetables.

Despite the fact that processed foods contain a significant quantity of fats and oils, the fats and oils found in these foods are not the healthiest forms to consume. What are the utmost daily allowances for fat, carbohydrates, protein, and cholesterol on the Dash diet?

Total fat - 27% 6% of calories are derived from saturated lipids

10 10 % of the total calories you consume originate from carbohydrates. 2 8% of the total calories you consume originate from protein. 2 10 0 milligrams of cholesterol are present in the diet.

A Catalog of Food

Following is a comprehensive list of foods and ingredients that you should be able to safely consume while adhering to the Dash diet if you are still having difficulty deciding what foods to purchase when you go grocery shopping.

Fruits & Vegetables:

Apples, artichokes, avocados, and berries are fruits and vegetables.

Bell Peppers, Broccoli Cabbage Carrots, Grapes Cauliflower Corn Cauliflower Green Beans, Lemons & Lime Squash The salad consists of Lettuce, Onions, Pears, Pineapple, Potatoes, Raisins, Sprouts, and Squash.

Both Meat and Marine Life:

Meat, Chicken, and Turkey Fresh eggs Aquatic and Seafood Shrimp and Salmon Bread, Cereals, Nuts, and Dairy Products:

Some Whole Wheat Products, Including Whole Wheat Bread and Tortillas Oats, Barley, and Brown Rice Wild Rice, Whole Wheat Pasta, and Whole-Grain Foods Cereal

Other Nuts and Seeds, Including Almonds, Cashews, Peanuts, and Others

Walnuts Pecans Pumpkin Seeds Pecans Lactic compounds.

Reduced-fat Cheeses, cottage cheese, and fat-free milk with margarine.

Purchasing Counsel

Important things to remember:

If you keep a few essential points in mind, grocery shopping while on the Dash diet can be an enjoyable and stress-free experience.

Before heading out to conduct your purchasing, you must first ensure that you are well-prepared. Create an inventory of the ingredients you'll need to prepare the meals you've planned for the next few days or week. Include all of the food you will need on the journey, including snacks and breakfast. Making a comprehensive list of everything you intend to consume in the coming days is the most effective method for saving money and sticking to your diet plan. If you do not have a list, it will be much simpler to deviate from your plan and consume items that are both tempting and unhealthy.

Do not visit the grocery store when you are extremely hungry. For your own health, consume something before going grocery shopping. Going to the grocery store when you're hungry is the surest way to fill your cart with unhealthy foods, since everything appears more enticing when you're hungry.

Don't overlook the Dash diet's fundamental principles.

The Dash diet emphasizes consuming primarily unprocessed and fresh foods. When you go grocery purchasing, prioritize freshness above all else. The fewer processing stages required, the better. This suggests that you should restrict your purchasing to the sections labeled "vegetable," "poultry and seafood," and "dairy." You should spend the majority of your time in the section containing fresh vegetables of various varieties. Fresh dishes are rich in essential nutrients such as vitamins and minerals, and also contain a substantial amount of fiber. When following the Dash diet, you should strive to accomplish all of these objectives. Avoid refrigerated foods, such as pizzas and lunch meats, as well as anything that is canned.

In most grocery stores, the fresh food sections are located along the store's perimeter. Always read the labeling. It is impossible to emphasize this point enough. The majority of Americans consume processed foods, but the vast majority have no idea what ingredients they contain. Acclimate yourself to spending the additional time necessary to peruse the label and become knowledgeable about the products you purchase. Typically, numerous products contain sodium that is not readily apparent. Consume exclusively low-sodium, low-fat, and low-calorie foods.

Stock your kitchen with Dash diet-compliant goods.

Because it is so versatile and can be substituted for less nutritious sweets, fruit is one of the most useful pantry essentials to always have on hand. Both snacking on fruits such as bananas, oranges, apples, and grapes and incorporating dried or unsweetened fruits into salads are healthful and tasty options.

It's not always simple to get people interested in vegetables, but given enough time, you'll discover that fresh salads are among their favorite foods. The key to effectively preparing vegetables is having a wide variety to choose from. The greater the variety, the more distinct flavors you will be able to enjoy. Having vegetables such as tomatoes, carrots, lettuce, mushrooms, broccoli, mixed greens, and spinach on hand in the kitchen is a fantastic method to ensure success with everyday cooking.

Your diet will likely include a substantial quantity of whole grains, and these grains and salad vegetables can pair very well. You should always stock your pantry with a variety of whole grains to accommodate a variety of preferences.

Whole grain meals include "brown rice" and "wild rice" in addition to "whole grain bread," "quinoa," "millet," "whole grain cereal," "oatmeal," and a variety of other cereals. Explore the various types of whole cereals.

On the Dash diet, legumes, seeds, and almonds will all play an important role in protein provision. There is an abundance of protein in legumes, such as kidney beans and navy beans. Lentils can be used to make a very substantial soup, and they are an excellent source of iron. Compared to nuts, which are also an excellent option, seeds such as sunflower seeds contain less total fat.

The inclusion of seeds and nuts to raw salads is incredibly beneficial. Whenever possible, it is essential to choose unsalted or low-salt versions of almonds and seeds.

You can meet your protein needs by consuming lean meats, fish, and poultry. It is advised that you restrict your diet to fish and poultry. Choose turkey or chicken without the skin. Fish contains relatively little natural fat. In addition to pork tenderloin, additional options include extra-lean minced beef and beef cuts such as round and sirloin.

On the Dash diet, low-fat dairy products such as low-fat or non-fat milk, low-fat cheese, yogurt, and sour cream are permitted. Additionally, you may consume low-fat kefir. Herbs, spices, flavored olive oils and vinegars, as well as flavored vinegars, are excellent substitutes for table salt because they impart flavor to food without the inclusion of salt.

Purchase some new cookware.

Using nonstick cookware when cooking meat or vegetables is an excellent way to reduce the quantity of oil or butter required. You can reduce the quantity of butter or oil you use by using a vegetable or rice steamer instead of a pot. The use of a garlic press or spice mill makes it much easier to enhance a dish's flavor without introducing additional salt.

Consider how to prepare food in a healthful manner.

Add a variety of seasonings and herbs, as well as garlic, ginger, lemon, flavored vinegar, and peppers, to enhance the flavor without adding sodium. It is essential to rinse canned vegetables, tomatoes, and tuna to simple Remove any excess sodium from the packing liquid.

The salt content of numerous broths can be quite significant. It is simple to make vegetable broth at home by sautéing vegetables such as mushrooms, shallots, and water. You may also find broths with minimal or no sodium in stores. Reduce the quantity of meat you consume. Initially, this may be difficult for you, but after some time, you will become acclimated to the various vegetarian meal options and realize you do not miss meat at all. You can reduce the quantity of meat in recipes by using only a portion of the total amount of meat called for in the recipe.

Chapter 7: What Does Dash Stand For?

DASH is an acronym for Dietary Approaches to Stop Hypertension. The DASH diet is not a passing fad, but rather a sustainable approach to healthy dieting. The purpose of this diet is to alter dietary habits in order to reduce hypertension, which can lead to fatal diseases and complications. Dietary Approaches to Stop Hypertension (DASH) is not a quick fix for weight loss, but rather a lifelong dietary plan that can be monitored and adhered to. My recipes utilize a variety of ingredients, so sacrificing flavor for health is not an issue.

The DASH diet treats and prevents hypertension by reducing sodium consumption and increasing dietary sources of potassium, magnesium, and calcium, which have been shown to reduce blood pressure. Not only does it reduce hypertension, but it also reduces your risk for osteoporosis, cardiovascular disease, and strokes. The DASH diet includes dinners that are rich in vegetables, organic products, and whole grains. In addition to these primary nutritional categories, the diet also includes small amounts of low-fat dairy, fish, poultry, and legumes.

What to Consume and Avoid

Now let's discuss which foods are permitted on the diet and which should be avoided. The portion sizes of healthful DASH diet meals throughout the day will also be examined. Keep in mind that the DASH diet is a lifelong adjustment, so do not restrict your diet; instead, make changes.

Good Foods to Consume

First, grains are essential to the DASH diet. This may include noodles, rice, oats, and bread. Grains are the foundation of your diet, so you should consume 6 to 8 servings per day. This varies depending on the individual, but for a typical 2,000-calorie diet, this is an appropriate serving size. One serving can consist of a slice of whole wheat bread, a cup of cooked pasta or rice, or one ounce of dried cereal.

The next largest nutritional category is vegetables. For a daily regimen of 2,000 calories, four to five servings of vegetables should be consumed. Vegetables rich in fiber and nutrients are exceptional for the DASH diet. Make your plate as vibrant as possible by combining vegetables of various hues. Try to incorporate leafy greens into your diet for an adequate amount of iron and protein. A substantial portion of one cup of cooked or raw vegetables equals one serving, whereas one cup of salad greens equals one serving.

Fruits are readily available and should be consumed at the same rate as vegetables. This means you are consuming four to five servings of delicious organic produce. High in fiber, potassium, magnesium, and other essential nutrients and minerals, natural products are essential to the DASH diet.

To increase the amount of fiber in your diet, don't peel a portion of your favorite organic fruits and vegetables, such as pears, before eating them. The epidermis is rich in dietary fibers.

Nuts, seeds, and vegetables should be consumed similarly to verdant greens. Aim for four to five daily servings of these super-pressed healthy food sources. They provide protein, potassium, magnesium, fiber, phytochemicals, and various additional nutrients. Various legumes, seeds, and nuts can be incorporated into your diet to meet these requirements. Low-fat or non-fat dairy products should account for no more than two to three of your daily servings. This may contain milk, cheddar cheese, or yogurt. When purchasing these items, we emphasize that they should be minimal in fat or fat-free. Dairy is included in the DASH diet to increase calcium, protein, and vitamin D, not to increase calories and fat.

The DASH diet allows poultry and fish, with a daily limit of six one-ounce servings. However, you should strive to consume primarily vegetables and to replace any meat in your diet with vegetables. If you choose to consume meat, avoid adding sodium and simple Remove the skin prior to consumption. Choose fish that are rich in omega-6 unsaturated fats when consuming fish. This can be fish such as salmon, which are exceptional for cardiac health.

Bad Foods to Consume

Now that we know what food sources are excellent to consume on the DASH diet and how many servings of each nutrition class we should consume, let's examine what food sources should be avoided on the DASH diet. In general, avoid consuming foods that are abundant in sugar, fat, and salt.

The DASH diet does not emphasize sweets. It is prescribed to consume no more than five desserts per week. Again, the DASH diet is not about depriving yourself of your favorite foods, but rather about consuming them with moderation. Therefore, the DASH diet permits you to consume these "cheat" foods in small amounts throughout the week. Alcohol has been shown to increase blood pressure. It is suggested that women consume approximately one beverage per day, while males consume approximately two per day. The wisest option is to abstain from alcohol entirely, but we recognize that occasional consumption is acceptable. If you find yourself consuming more than you should each evening, try removing all alcoholic beverages from your home. Thus, you can consume it on a night out while preventing easy access from the container. Red meat should be avoided or consumed infrequently on the DASH diet. Both red meat's elevated fat and sodium content are detrimental to the DASH diet. If you're looking for flesh, stick to poultry or lean pork. Full-fat dairy products, such as heavy whipping cream and 2% milk, should be avoided. This increases the number of fat servings you consume per day, and in order to stay on the DASH diet, you must ensure that your fat servings consistently register. Be wary of beverages. Numerous beverages, comparable to soda, contain high levels of sugar and artificial sugars. Abstain from imbibing these and instead obtain your sugar intake from satiating food sources. Consume your calories rather than imbibing them.

Due to the manner in which fast food is prepared, it is typically high in sodium and should be avoided. This includes crackers, pizza, and other unhealthy snacks. They can also conceal carbohydrates added to enhance the food's flavor, whereas the nutritional value is diminished.

The DASH diet emphasizes mindful nutrition. You are responsible for selecting food sources that nourish and energize you rather than harm you.

Remember these portion sizes and nutrient groups when preparing your next DASH diet meal.

Q AND A

You should now have a well-rounded understanding of the DASH diet. You are aware of the portions and types of food you should consume, the food sources to avoid, and the benefits of the DASH diet. Nonetheless, if you have any lingering concerns, here are some answers and tips to keep in mind as you embark on your journey to better health.

How challenging is it to comply with the DASH diet?

Answer: The DASH diet is not comparable to other eating plans from which you may fall off due to food variety restriction. Because the DASH diet incorporates a variety of food sources, you will not become exhausted from adhering to a conventionally stringent and restrictive diet. As a result, the DASH diet is not a quick fix for weight loss, but rather a lifestyle modification that promotes long-term health. With increasing levels of obesity on the planet. The DASH diet is a way to check these statistics without sacrificing your preferred food sources. As a result, the diet allows for 10 servings of sugar per week, recognizing that these cravings will inevitably arise and that moderate consumption is the most effective method for managing them.

Where would I be able to purchase food for my DASH consume less carbs diet?

Do I really intend to purchase dietary supplements or pills?

The reason the DASH diet is so effective is that it is flexible. Under DASH guidelines, you may purchase all of the ingredients for any recipe from a supermarket, farmers market, health food store, or wherever you choose to purchase your food. There are no additional enhancements or security measures required to purchase online repairs. This regimen consists of only you, another list of staple foods, and a trip to the market.

Are you interested in adopting the DASH diet?

Answer: Exercise is not required to reap the health benefits of the DASH diet. Regardless, exercise in conjunction with a healthy diet can improve your health. Cardio along with strength training can help you consume more calories, lose weight, and achieve your health objectives faster. Similarly, practice does not need to be extensive. You can commence with as little as 6 0 minutes of daily walking.

If my heart rate is normal, would it be wise for me to adopt the DASH diet? The DASH diet is designed to reduce circulatory distress in individuals with hypertension. If you already have high blood pressure, this diet may not be the best option for you. Dietary principles, such as consuming more vegetables and avoiding red meat, are beneficial for everyone. The diet eventually focuses on smart dieting, which is a good illustration for individuals with or without hypertension. Those with a rapid heart rate, however, would benefit more from a diet that is more tailored to their specific needs. Consult with your primary care physician (PCP) or other specialists about various options for smart, long-term diet plans that are suitable for you.

Chapter 8: Contras To The Dash Diet Weight Loss

The DASH diet was originally designed to assist individuals in lowering their blood pressure. As an additional bonus, scientists discovered that healthy eating also resulted in weight loss. If you are looking to lose weight, there may be a healthier diet out there for you. Please bear in mind that although there are diets designed for weight loss, there is a reason why many people regain the weight. Most regimens are intended for temporary weight loss. The DASH diet is intended for lifelong consumption. As you can see from our list of advantages, the DASH diet is quite flexible. If you wish to lose weight, you must merely consume fewer calories. There are far too many benefits you would lose out on if you chose not to follow the DASH diet solely because it was not initially designed for weight loss.

Support System

The DASH diet appears to be an independent regimen. No appointed groups are intended to guide you through your new lifestyle. If you are the type of person who requires regular meetings and social support, this regimen may not be for you. The DASH diet will require you to be your own support system. You must remind yourself that you are acting in your own best interest. Remind yourself that you are attempting to lose weight or improve your health for a specific purpose. There is always the possibility of forming your own group, but you would have to do so on your own leisure. In fact, we encourage you to form a support group if you believe it will help you persevere. Bring along your family and close acquaintances. We are confident that as soon as you begin the DASH diet, becoming healthier and possibly even losing weight, they will be inquiring how you did it!

Absence of convenience

Perhaps you are the sort of person who requires the door-to-door delivery of prepackaged foods. In this circumstance, the DASH diet is not appropriate for you.

Unfortunately for those averse to take the time to cook, these foods are not available in the freezer section already prepared. We acknowledge that this diet will require a bit more of your time and effort. This work will be well worth it in the end, because you deserve it. Regarding your diet, it is all about your mental state. You could view the foods as a significant inconvenience, or you could be grateful for the ability to purchase fresh foods and fuel your body to its maximum capacity. You can alter both your mindset and your lifestyle simultaneously!

Food Selections

While some may view this as a drawback of any diet, we assure you that a diet change does not have to be monotonous! When you hear the word "diet," the thought of giving up your beloved foods may make you sad. As an indulgence, some of us require chocolate or ice cream. We assure you that consuming kale for the remainder of your life is not a consequence of your diet. While you may be reducing your consumption of processed foods and meaningless carbohydrates, we do not prohibit you from consuming anything. It is all about moderation and discretion. As you will discover in later chapters, these are merely recommendations. You may adhere to the DASH diet however you wish, but keep in mind that the effort you put in will determine the outcome. Yes, we encourage you to indulge in that sweet treat because life is brief. However, everything must be done in moderation. It is a rule that everyone should adhere to in various aspects of their lives. This change in culinary options should not be viewed negatively; instead, it should be greeted with open arms. The recipes that follow will demonstrate that healthy eating can be exceedingly delicious. In addition, you will be improving your health simultaneously. What could go wrong?

Chapter 9: What Is The Dash Diet?

The DASH diet is very convenient and requires little time for food selection and preparation. High-cholesterol and saturated fat-containing foods should be tolerated. The individual is encouraged to consume as many vegetables, fruits, and grains as feasible.

In order to prevent sagging of the intestines and other stomach-related maladies, it is concluded that the consumption of high-fiber foods should be restricted in gradual increments when following the DASH diet. You can progressively increase your fiber intake by consuming an extra portion of leafy vegetables with each meal. Cereals are an additional excellent source of fiber, B vitamins, and minerals. To increase your fiber consumption, you can consume whole grains, whole wheat bread, bran, wheat germ, and low-fat breakfast cereals.

You can select the foods you consume by reading the labels on prepared and packaged foods. Consider consuming foods that are low in fat, sodium, and cholesterol. Meats, chocolate, french fries, and fast food are the primary sources of fat and cholesterol, so you should limit your consumption of these foods.

If you want to consume meat but limit your daily intake to six ounces, which is equivalent to playing cards, you can incorporate more vegetables, cereals, pasta, and beans into your meat dishes. Additionally, skim or skim milk is a source of high-quality protein devoid of excess fat and cholesterol. As an alternative to munchies, you may choose canned or dried fruit, as well as fresh fruit.

DASH diet guidelines

You are aware that the DASH diet is a nutritional plan that emphasizes the consumption of fresh, high-quality, and lean proteins and adheres to the guidelines of the United States Food Pyramid. Any diet centered on these foods is bound to be successful, so what is it about the DASH diet that makes it so beneficial and one of the best diets physicians recommend? The DASH diet not only considers the overall health of foods, but also goes beyond nutrient content, including calcium, potassium, and magnesium. This ensures that you receive a daily combination of nutritional components that promote the highest possible level of health in your body. What to consume while following the DASH diet plan is outlined below. These recommendations are based on a daily caloric intake of 2 ,800 to 2,000 calories. The number of calories you consume will depend on your current body type, level of physical activity, and whether weight loss or overall health improvement is your primary objective. Numerous factors are considered when determining an individual's optimal calorie intake.

Therefore, it is recommended to consult a physician or other qualified professional who is familiar with your situation. Adjust these portions according to your desired daily caloric intake. Also, bear in mind that during phase one of the DASH diet, consumption of grains and fruits is restricted, whereas phase two of the plan follows the guidelines for these food groups. Activity level and whether or not weight loss or overall health improvement is your primary objective. Numerous factors are considered when determining an individual's optimal calorie intake.

Therefore, it is recommended to consult a physician or other qualified professional who is familiar with your situation. Adjust these portions according to your desired daily caloric intake. Also, bear in mind that during phase one of the DASH diet, consumption of grains and fruits is restricted, whereas phase two of the plan follows the guidelines for these food groups. Activity level and whether or not weight loss or overall health improvement is your primary objective. Numerous factors are considered when determining an individual's optimal calorie intake.

Therefore, it is recommended to consult a physician or other qualified professional who is familiar with your situation. Adjust these portions according to your desired daily caloric intake. Also, bear in mind that during phase one of the DASH diet, consumption of grains and fruits is restricted, whereas phase two of the plan follows the guidelines for these food groups. It is best to discuss this with a doctor or other qualified professional who can be considerate of your circumstances. Adjust these portions according to your desired daily caloric intake. Also, observe that during phase one of the DASH diet, consumption of grains and fruits is restricted, whereas phase two of the plan follows the suggested guidelines for these food groups. It is best to discuss this with a doctor or other qualified professional who can be considerate of your circumstances. Adjust these portions according to your desired daily caloric intake.

Is the DASH diet the best choice for you?

DASH diet is an outstanding plan for everyone.

The prevalence of metabolic syndrome is rising due to the increasing prevalence of morbid obesity in the United States and elsewhere. If you are significantly overweight or overweight and have excess abdominal fat, you may have metabolic syndrome or develop it.

The best aspect is that metabolic syndrome can be reversed in whole or in part by combining physical activity and a DASH-style diet. Experts have discovered that individuals with type two diabetes can achieve comparable outcomes.

But what if none of these diseases affect you? What if you're simply looking for a healthy method to lose weight and potentially prevent these conditions in the future?

If you are contemplating the DASH diet for weight loss and prevention, you are more likely to view it as a desirable long-term health option. The DASH diet recommends consuming a broad variety of foods from all food groups, will guide you through the process of determining your ideal calorie intake, and will typically improve participants' metabolism and energy levels. While many other diet plans promote unhealthy eating habits and deprivation, the DASH diet-based nutritional approach is a practical and excellent choice for many.

Additional benefits of the DASH diet include: • You are more likely to find

DASH-friendly meals when dining out or at a friend's house; • The realistic forms of DASH ensure that it is easier to maintain the weight once you have reached your ideal weight; • You can choose the sodium level that is right for you; and • The DASH eating pattern explains how you can increase or decrease calorie intake as your activity level and body mass change.

• It is simple to adapt familiar dishes to the DASH Diet.

It is not difficult to understand why millions of people have considered adopting the DASH diet to lose weight and enhance their health. This guide provides everything necessary for a successful meal.

How to better initiate the second phase of meals in Chapter 2.

There are two phases to the DASH diet: phase one and phase two. The initial phase is the rapid-start phase, which attempts to restore your metabolism. This phase is protein-rich and sugar- and carbohydrate-restrictive. This phase of the diet typically lasts for the first two weeks, giving your body time to adapt to the new eating habits. Since this is a 2 8 - day all-inclusive plan, we have shortened this phase to the first seven days, and then we will introduce phase two, which consists of fresh produce, pulses, and cereals. During period 2 , you will consume greater quantities of lean meats, low-fat dairy products, and nuts than were initially recommended. This is to ensure that you consume sufficient calories and a variety of foods during this phase. You can extend it to a 22 -day plan if you wish, and you can prolong aspect one in two weeks by simply repeating it. Alternately, if you do not desire to participate in phase one and would rather begin period two for health benefits that do not include rapid initial weight loss, you may do so. Continue directly to phase two and repeat for two weeks. If you do not wish to participate in phase one and would rather begin phase two for health benefits other than rapid initial weight loss, this is also acceptable. Continue directly to phase two and repeat for two weeks. If you do not wish to participate in phase one and would rather begin phase two for health benefits other than rapid initial weight loss, this is also acceptable. Continue directly to phase two and repeat for two weeks.

This regimen is based on a daily caloric intake between 2 800 and 2000 calories and is designed to provide you with all of the essential nutrients. If weight loss is your primary objective, a health care professional may recommend cutting calories in one way or another. Keep in mind that Phase One's high protein and carbohydrate content allows you to consume more calories while still losing weight. The objective is to increase your metabolism, not to inhibit it by severely restricting your caloric intake.

A few items to remember throughout the 2 8 -day plan: Initially, substitutions are permitted. It is not a regimen in which you are required to consume specific foods without deviation. It is a change in lifestyle, and it should suit your lifestyle. This will not occur if you attempt to consume unpalatable foods or skip meals and snacks to prevent them. The DASH diet emphasizes calcium-, magnesium-, and potassium-rich foods.

If you are replacing a food, the only rule is that the replacement food must have a similar nutritional profile, particularly for these three nutrients. In light of this, studies have demonstrated that we derive the most benefit from nutrients when we obtain them from their dietary sources rather than as supplements. If you are food intolerant or unable to consume certain foods, it is permissible to take supplements.

The DASH diet has been designed to combat factors that can lead to straightforward complications. Some of these factors, such as sodium and cholesterol, have already been mentioned. The remaining factors will be covered in subsequent chapters of the book. It is crucial to note that the DASH diet is not an all-encompassing approach. You need persistence, perseverance, and dedication to achieve your objective. Beginning this endeavor requires motivation and determination, but it won't be too difficult if you follow these straightforward instructions.

2 . Take your time.

If this diet is unexpected, do not despair. You are not required to embrace it immediately. Proceed if you are satisfied with the application in a step-by-step process. Due to the numerous components of this diet, it is impossible to implement them all at once. You can begin with your sodium consumption. If you enjoy salted foods, it's time to reduce your intake, but you don't have to do so immediately. If your daily sodium intake is ten tablespoons, which is significantly higher than what is recommended, you can reduce it to nine tablespoons immediately. You can presumably try this for a week, then reduce the dosage by one tablespoon per day the following week.

The same holds true if you dislike consuming vegetables and are gluttonous. You can introduce one vegetable at a time until you become accustomed to it.

2. Replace.

Currently, a variety of foods are available for purchase and can be substituted for harmful alternatives. If you enjoy drinking milk in the morning or evening and do not wish to reduce your consumption, consider low-fat or fat-free dairy products. Other dairy products, such as cheese and butter, now have reduced-fat alternatives. Consider them. These products help reduce blood cholesterol levels. Try herbs like rosemary, basil, and thyme for a flavorful dish without sodium. They make your cuisine both delicious and nutritious.

6 . Remove.

The second-best option is to examine your kitchen, particularly your refrigerator, for healthy and harmful foods. According to the Hypertension principles and the DASH diet, which substances should be eliminated immediately? Maintain the leanness of your vegetables, fruits, and meat; eliminate sugary, greasy, and salty foods. This removes future temptations to consume toxic foods. From that point on, you can plan your meals with healthful eating in mind only.

Develop a meal schedule.

To facilitate adoption of the DASH diet, it is preferable to have a meal plan prepared and adhere to it. Plan enough meals for breakfast, lunch, supper, and snacks over the course of the week to guide your food consumption. It also helps you maintain a balanced diet. Plan a meal consisting of cereals, fruits and vegetables, fish and meat, and limit sugary and fattening foods.

10 . Make a list.

When purchasing ingredients, it is recommended to have a shopping list based on your meal plan. Be devoted to your list. This helps you avoid purchasing expensive and harmful foods that will only increase your grocery bill

and take up too much space in your
refrigerator.

Chapter 10: Understanding The Dash Diet's Foundational Elements

The DASH diet is founded on a combination of nutrients known to influence blood pressure, such as:

Fruits, vegetables, and whole cereals are rich in fiber, potassium, and other minerals that lower blood pressure.

Low-fat dairy products: Milk, cheese, and yogurt are abundant in calcium and protein, which can help reduce blood pressure.

Low in saturated fat and cholesterol, lean protein sources consist of lean meats, poultry, fish, legumes, and tofu.

Nuts, seeds, and legumes are rich in fiber, protein, and other nutrients that lower blood pressure.

These lipids and sugars have been shown to raise blood pressure.

The DASH diet also incorporates sodium intake guidelines, as a high sodium intake can contribute to high blood pressure. The DASH diet recommends limiting daily sodium intake to 2,6 00 milligrams or less, with an option to go as low as 2 ,10 00 milligrams for individuals with severe hypertension or a high risk of heart disease.

Dietary Approaches to Stop Hypertension (DASH) is a healthful eating pattern that emphasizes whole, minimally processed foods and encourages the consumption of a variety of nutrients known to have a positive effect on blood pressure. It is an age-appropriate, well-balanced diet suitable for those with high blood pressure or who are at risk for developing it.

The main components of the DASH diet are:

Emphasis on fruits, vegetables, and whole grains: The DASH diet recommends consuming a large quantity of fruits, vegetables, and whole grains, as these foods are rich in nutrients that can help lower blood pressure.

Sodium restriction: The DASH diet recommends consuming no more than 2,6 00 milligrams (mg) of sodium per day, and preferably less. A high sodium intake has been associated with high blood pressure, so limiting your sodium intake can help to lower your blood pressure.

Consuming low-fat dairy products: The DASH diet suggests consuming low-fat or fat-free dairy products because they are lower in saturated fat and cholesterol, which can help reduce blood pressure.

Limiting consumption of saturated and total fats: The DASH diet recommends limiting consumption of saturated and total fats, as these forms of fat have been associated with high blood pressure.

The DASH diet encourages the consumption of lean protein sources, such as chicken, turkey, salmon, beans, and nuts, because they are lower in saturated fat and cholesterol.

Maintain a healthy weight and blood pressure by consuming meals and refreshments on a regular basis.

Stay hydrated: Consume copious amounts of water throughout the day to eliminate excess sodium from your system.

Remember that the DASH diet is not a fast weight loss solution. It is a long-term, healthy eating plan that can help reduce high blood pressure and enhance overall health. Consult a healthcare professional if you have any specific queries or concerns about the DASH diet or your health.

Overall, the DASH diet is a heart-healthy eating plan that focuses on lowering blood pressure through the consumption of nutrient-rich foods and the restriction of certain nutrients linked to high blood pressure.

Chapter 11: How To Maintain The Weight Loss Achieved Using These Methods

Weight loss is a prevalent objective for many individuals. Losing weight and maintaining a healthy weight will help you minimize specific problems, have more energy, and feel better in general. However, there are numerous diet programs for sale that are extremely complicated or extremely expensive. Therefore, devising a weight loss plan that you can maintain over the long term will be significantly more beneficial. Adapt this program to your lifestyle by considering the potential costs, the aspects of dieting you enjoy or detest, and the frequency of physical activity. Remember these aspects.

Create a plan for weight loss.

Schedule an appointment with your physician. Consult your physician to determine your ideal weight and the number of pounds you should lose. In addition, the professional will evaluate any medications you take and any illnesses you may have in order to determine if it is safe for you to begin a weight loss program.

Your physician will also assist you in determining if your physical condition allows you to engage in strenuous regimens or exercises.

In addition, he will provide you with essential tips for calorie counting and determining what is ideal for you.

Set achievable objectives Every time you begin a (bought or owned) weight loss program, it is vital to establish reasonable objectives. This will help you determine the type of diet, duration, and (if necessary) physical activity to perform. In general, individuals who set themselves overly ambitious goals become discouraged or lose motivation, and ultimately give up. Put the plan on the calendar to motivate yourself to follow through.

It is not generally advised to lose more than 0.10 to 2 kilogram (2 to 2 pounds) per week. Considered to be secure, realistic, and sustainable for weight loss.

Diets that promise more rapid and substantial weight loss are typically unsafe and unsustainable. Focus instead on simpler, more attainable objectives.

Set yourself multiple objectives if you need to lose several pounds. You can have both a long-term objective and shorter-term objectives. For instance, a long-term objective could be to lose 2 10 pounds (6 0 pounds) in six months. Short-term objectives may include losing 2.10 kilograms (10 pounds) in two weeks, 10 kilograms (2 0 pounds) in four or five weeks, etc.

Purchase or create a calendar for goal tracking. Underline the beginning and ending dates of the program. In this manner, you will establish a deadline for attaining your objectives, thereby paving the way forward.

Additionally, you can specify the days you desire to exercise. Ensure that they are noted on the calendar.

Place the calendar in a prominent location so that you can always see it and remember your obligations. If this indicates that you should engage in cardiovascular exercise, then do so.

Create a system of rewards. Determining desirable rewards will keep you motivated throughout the duration of the program. Ensure that these are specific, one-of-a-kind activities that you will only book when you reach your target.

Define smaller rewards as incentives for accomplishing smaller intermediate objectives. When you achieve larger, longer-term objectives, you should reward yourself with a larger bonus.

In general, it is not recommended that rewards be tied to food (such as dining out or purchasing a dessert). Choose rewards that are unrelated to food, such as a manicure, new clothes or shoes, a massage, a round of golf at your favored course, or a new book.

Plan for lifestyle modifications. It is advisable to avoid fad regimens whenever you are attempting to lose weight. Instead, adopt a lifelong healthier lifestyle.

Small dietary and lifestyle modifications are simpler to maintain over time. You should avoid making drastic adjustments when losing weight, as it is unlikely that you will be able to maintain them.

Create a plan for weight loss.

Set a daily calorie restriction. Whatever weight-loss program you choose, it will inevitably reduce calories to achieve your objectives. Determine the daily caloric intake required to lose 0.10 to 2 kilogram (2 to 2 pounds) per week.

In general, to lose 0.10 to 2 kg (2 to 2 pounds), you will need to reduce your caloric intake, increase your caloric expenditure, or plan a combination of the two to remove and expend between 10 00 and 2 000 calories per day.

First, determine how many calories you consume on an average day when you're not dieting. You can use an app or an online calculator to determine the number of calories you consume each day. Subtract between 10 00 and 700 calories from this number to determine approximately how many calories you need to consume.

On the Internet, you can also find calculators and mobile applications that calculate the number of calories you must consume to lose weight based on your age, gender, current weight, and level of physical activity.

Calculate the portions. In order to maintain a low-calorie diet, it is crucial to consider the appropriate portion sizes for meals and snacking. If you serve or consume large portions, losing weight will be difficult for you.

Purchase a kitchen scale or measuring containers to avoid overdosing. Measurement of each meal and snack to assure compliance with dietary restrictions.

Purchase specific-sized containers, bowls, platters, and cups to facilitate the process. For instance, you can preserve your lunch in a container that contains a cup of food.

There exists a suitable portion measurement for most meals. In general, you should consume 6 to 8 ounces (810 to 2 2 0 grams) of protein, 1 cup of cut fruit or a small portion of fruit, 2 to 2 cups of green leafy vegetables, and 6 0 to 6 10 milligrams of grain. cup

Plan a diet high or moderate in protein. Depending on your preference, you will need to choose between a high or medium protein diet. This is the key to creating a meal plan you can adhere to without going hungry.

Several studies have demonstrated that high-protein diets promote weight loss and weight maintenance.

Consuming a portion of lean protein with each meal and refreshment is optimal for any weight loss plan. If you are following a high protein diet, you may need to consume more than one serving per meal.

Consider a protein-rich cuisine if you've been very hungry on your previous diets. It has been shown that consuming more protein throughout the day results in a greater sense of satiety.

Try a diet low or moderate in carbs. Meal plans are typically divided into two categories: low-carbohydrate diets and moderate-carbohydrate diets. Both options have benefits; choose the one that best fits your lifestyle.

Low-carb diets have been shown to facilitate weight loss more rapidly than moderate-nutrient diets. However, both regimens have produced comparable weight loss results overall.

Diets low in carbohydrates are more restricting. This could be the correct diet for you if it is simple for you and you do not lack carbohydrates.

Some individuals are extremely apprehensive about carbohydrate consumption, while others believe that incorporating a moderate quantity of carbs each day yields superior results. Again, select the alternative that best suits your requirements and way of life.

If you choose to restrict your carbohydrate intake, begin by limiting your cereal group options (bread, white rice, pasta, crackers, etc.). This food group contains few nutrients that cannot be derived from other sources. Limit your intake of starchy foods (beans, potatoes, winter squash, and peas) if you wish to adopt a low-carbohydrate diet.

Include vegetables and fruits in your diet. There are numerous dietary patterns available. The majority, however, consists of daily consumption of multiple portions of fruits and vegetables.

Both fruits and vegetables are low in calories and extremely nutritious. They are rich in numerous vitamins, minerals, antioxidants, and fiber.

Consume no more than one or two portions of produce per day. If you wish to adhere to a low-carb diet, you should consume less food.

Consume roughly five servings of vegetables per day. Again, if you wish to adhere to a low-carb diet, select starchy vegetables over high-carb vegetables (such as potatoes, peas, and carrots).

Consume hydrating liquids daily. Taking into consideration the adequate consumption of water and other hydrating liquids is an essential aspect of developing a plan for weight loss. This will enable you to control your appetite and improve your overall health.

A decent starting point is to consume eight glasses of water per day. This may necessitate up to 2 6 beverages per day. The precise quantity will depend on your gender, weight, and physical activity level.

Purchase a bottle of water to keep track of the amount of fluids you consume daily.

Include physical activity in your daily routine. It is essential to implement daily physical activity into your routine if you

165

wish to lose weight. Changing your diet and beginning a physical business at the same time can be quite overwhelming. If at all feasible, make one change at a time.

Regular physical activity promotes weight loss and long-term maintenance, according to a number of studies.

Consider the possibility of beginning a supervised or commercial diet. You may begin a business or supervised diet if you do not wish to construct your own meal plan. Additionally, you can base your strategy on one of the following:

A diet high in protein and low in carbohydrates. Some commercial programs are founded on a profile that is low in carbohydrates and high in protein.

In general, this type of diet produces rapid results, but its restrictive nature makes it difficult to maintain over time.

Low-fat diet This regimen intends to restrict the fat content of food. In particular, the majority of low-fat diets restrict the consumption of trans and saturated fats while permitting the consumption of heart-healthy lipids.

Mediterranean diet. This diet consists primarily of fruits, vegetables, whole grains, fish, and small quantities of beef or poultry protein. It has been shown to be a healthful option for individuals with heart problems and can prevent heart disease.

Learn more about weight loss medical programs. Dietary regimens are formulated by health professionals and dietitians. In general, these diets involve following a restrictive meal plan or ingesting low-calorie and high-protein substitutes for a brief period of time. In addition, you may require prescription medications, vitamin supplements, or injections to help suppress your appetite and boost your vitality.

Maintain a healthy weight over time.

Several studies have demonstrated that individuals who adhere to their meal plan tend to be more diet-conscious and to maintain their results over time. Regardless of your diet, recording your meals will increase your likelihood of success.

In addition, you can monitor your progress. Record your weekly weight and cumulative weight loss.

You may also document what works and what does not. When reevaluating the plan, reread the accompanying notes and make any necessary adjustments.

Reevaluate the plan monthly. Whether you're on a commercial diet or working on a personal endeavor, it's essential to evaluate your progress frequently. This will enable you to determine if the plan is suitable for you.

Evaluate the weight loss by weighing yourself weekly and calculating the total pounds lost during the month. If the results are favorable, you can proceed with the same strategy. If you have not lost a significant amount of weight, you should reread your food journal and calorie count to make the necessary adjustments.

Evaluate how simple it was to adhere to the plan. Did your meals satisfy your physical needs? Are you ravenous all day? Do you have significant anxiety and the desire to eat? Adapt the plan as necessary.

Establish a support group. Find a support group if you are attempting to reduce weight and keep it off permanently so that you can live a healthy lifestyle. A support group will help you maintain your weight loss over time.

Numerous studies have demonstrated that individuals who are part of a support group or who are in the company of friends, family, or even other dieters are more successful and have maintained their weight loss over time.

Discuss your new diet with your peers, family, neighbors, and coworkers. Inquire if they wish to enroll.

You can also locate support groups online. Find a group that holds personal meetings if you prefer.

Advice

Some individuals dislike the flavor of water. If this is the case, add lemon or lime slices to the water to enhance its flavor. In this manner, you will also reap the benefits of vitamin C.

Check each item you place in your shopping cart at the supermarket and ask yourself, "Will this help me lose weight?" If the answer is negative, return the item to the shelve.

If you are too occupied to exercise, incorporate physical activity into your obligations and activities. If you must visit a supermarket, attempt to do so at the closest location and purchase only what you require. If you must drive to a meeting in the city, arrive a little earlier than anticipated; park a few blocks away and take the stairs rather than the elevator.

Weight yourself daily. This will help you stay on track and monitor your progress.

However, remember that daily weight gain can differ between 2 and 2 kilograms. Therefore, you should not be shocked if the numbers fluctuate.

Pumpkin Soup

Ingredients:

- 2 small chopped onion

- ¼ cup water, divided

- 4 cups vegetable broth, unsalted

- 20 -ounce can pumpkin puree

- 1 teaspoon nutmeg, ground

- 2 cup milk, fat-free

- 1 teaspoon cinnamon, ground

- 2 chopped green onion top

- 1/7 teaspoon black pepper

1. In a saucepan over medium heat, heat ¼ cup water.

2. Add the onion and easy cook for about 5-10 minutes, until it becomes tender.

3. Also, don't dry out the onion.

4. Add the pumpkin, remaining water, broth, nutmeg, and cinnamon.

5. Boil the mixture.

6. Reduce the heat and simmer for mixture for 5-10 minutes.

7. Add in the milk and easy cook it further, but don't let the mixture boil.

8. Into warmed bowls, ladle the soup and garnish each serving with green onion tops and black pepper.

9. Serve immediately. Serves 8 .

Turkey Bean Soup

Ingredients:

- 2 minced garlic clove

- 6 cubes chicken bouillon, low sodium

- 2 2 8 .10 -ounce can diced tomatoes, unsalted

- 2 1 teaspoons basil, dried

- 14 cups water

- 4 cups cabbage, shredded

- 2 pound turkey breast, ground

- 4 stalks chopped celery

- 4 chopped medium onions

- ½ cup ketchup

- ½ teaspoon black pepper, ground

- 2 2 10 -ounce can cannellini beans, unsalted

1. In a saucepan, easy cook the onion, ground turkey, celery, and garlic until the turkey is cooked and the vegetables become soft.

2. Add the tomatoes, water, bouillon, ketchup, pepper, basil, beans, and cabbage.

3. Bring the mixture to boil and reduce the heat.

4. Cover the pot and simmer further for 60 minutes.

Omelet With Broccoli And Cheese

Number of Servings: 2

Ingredients:

- 1 cup chopped broccoli, steamed
- Ground turmeric
- Olive oil cooking spray
- 4 fresh egg whites
- 2 fresh egg
- 4 slices low fat pepper Jack cheese, torn

How to Prepare:

1. Whisk the fresh egg whites and fresh egg with a dash of turmeric in a bowl and set aside.

2. Coat a nonstick skillet with olive oil cooking spray and place over medium flame.

3. Pour the fresh egg mixture into the skillet and easy cook for 25 to 30 seconds, then add the broccoli. Flip over and sprinkle the cheese on top.

4. Easy cook for an additional 25 to 30 seconds, or until the fresh egg is set to a desired level of consistency and the cheese is melted.

5. Transfer the omelet onto a plate, slice in half, and serve at once.

Nutty Banana Pancakes

Ingredients:

- 4 teaspoons of oil
- 6 large fresh egg whites
- 4 tablespoons of chopped walnuts
- 2 teaspoon of vanilla
- 4 teaspoons of baking powder
- 2 cup of whole wheat flour
- ½ teaspoon of cinnamon
- ½ teaspoon of salt
- 2 cup of 2 % milk
- 2 large banana, mashed

Directions:

1. Mix together the baking powder, flour, cinnamon, salt, and walnuts.

2. Combine the mashed bananas, vanilla, oil, fresh egg white, and milk in a separate bowl until smooth.

3. Pour the banana mixture into the flour mixture and mix together until well-combined.

4. Be careful not to over-mix.

5. Set a large pan over medium heat. Lightly coat the pan with cooking spray.

6. Pour ½ cup of batter and easy cook until it starts to bubble.

7. Flip and easy cook the other side.

8. Do the same procedure with the remaining batter.

Stir-Fried Broccoli and Chicken Skip Chinese and enjoy this healthy and hearty meal with the whole family.

Serves 8

Ingredients:

- 12 oz of frozen snow peas
- 4 cups of frozen broccoli florets
- 4 cups of cooked brown rice
- 4 cups of shredded cabbage
- 2 tablespoon of sesame seeds
- 2 tablespoon of low sodium soy sauce
- 2 /6 cup of orange juice
- 4 teaspoons of cornstarch
- 2 tablespoon of Szechuan sauce
- 2 lb of boneless chicken breast, cubed to 2 -inch pieces
- 2 tablespoon of canola oil

Directions:

1.	Combine the cornstarch, Szechuan sauce, soy sauce, and orange juice in a small bowl.

2.	Add the canola oil in a wok. Once the oil is hot, add in the chicken and stir fry for 10 to 15 minutes.

3. Add in the snow peas, broccoli, cabbage, and the sauce mixture. Stir fry for 5-10 minutes.

4.	Serve on top of the brown rice. Sprinkle sesame seeds on top.

simple Remove Easy cook Simple Remove _

Gazpacho flavored with Mint Ingredients

- 2 teaspoon lemon juice

- 2 teaspoon lime juice

- 2 teaspoon lemon zest

- Fresh mint leaves for garnish

- 8 scoops yogurt

- 2 1 cups blueberries

- 2 1 cups raspberries

- 4 tablespoons raw sugar

- 2 tablespoon orange juice

Instructions

1. Mix berries, sugar, orange, lemon and lime juice and the lemon zest in a bowl.

2. Cover tightly with plastic wrap.

3. Place the covered bowl over a large saucepan of simmering water and easy cook on low 20 minutes.

4. Refrigerate for about 1-5 hours.

5. Divide fruit and its liquid among 5-10 bowls; garnish with fresh mint and top each bowl with a 1/2 cup scoop of yogurt.

Pumpkin-Cookies For Breakfast

Ingredients

- 2 tablespoon baking powder

- 2 1 teaspoons pumpkin pie spice mix

- 1 teaspoon salt

- 2 cup raisins

- 2 cup walnuts (chopped)

- 2 ¾ cups pureed pumpkin (cooked)

- 2 1 cups brown sugar

- 4 fresh eggs

- 1 cup vegetable oil

- 2 1 cups flour

- 3 cups whole wheat flour

Instructions

1. Preheat oven to 450 degrees F.

2. Mix pumpkin, brown sugar, fresh eggs, and oil in a bowl

3. Blend dry ingredients and add to pumpkin mixture.

4. Add raisins and nuts.

5. Drop by teaspoonful's on greased cookie sheet

6. Bake for 15 to 20 minutes until golden brown.

Breakfast Fruit Parfait

Ingredients

- 5-10 cups light fat-free vanilla yogurt

- 2 cup granola, crumbled

- 8 cups mixed strawberries and blueberries

Make

1. Place 1/2 cup of yogurt into each of the 1-5 juice or parfait glasses.

2. Add a layer of 1 cup berries then 4 tablespoons of granola.

3. Add another 1/2 cup of yogurt, then half a cup of the berries and then 4 tablespoons of crumbled granola.

4. Chill or serve immediately.

Blueberry Pancakes

Ingredients:

½ tsp. baking soda

½ tsp. baking powder

4 cups whole wheat flour

¼ tsp. sea salt

½ cup steel cut oats

5 cups water

1 cup Agave nectar

4 cups blueberries (frozen)

½ cup Greek yogurt (vanilla flavor)

4 cups milk

4 fresh eggs

Directions:

1. In a large pot, bring water to a boil.

2. Add sea salt and steel cut oats.

3. Reduce the heat and simmer for 25 to 30 minutes or until the oats becomes tender.

4. Simple Remove from heat and set aside for 35 to 40 minutes.

5. In a medium bowl meanwhile, combine yogurt, milk, fresh egg, baking soda, baking powder and whole wheat flour.

6. Mix until a batter forms.

7. Fold in the cooked oats and blueberries.

8. In a non-stick skillet, spray cooking oil then pour 1 of pancake batter.

9. Easy cook until a bubble appears.

10. Fold each sides and easy cook again until golden brown.

11. Garnish with agave nectar and serve.

Mimi's Lentil Stir-Fry **Ingredients**

- 1 cup rice vinegar
- 1/2 cup minced fresh mint
- 6 tablespoons olive oil
- 4 teaspoons honey
- 2 teaspoon dried basil
- 2 teaspoon dried oregano
- 8 cups fresh baby spinach, chopped
- 2 cup (8 ounces) crumbled feta cheese
- 8 bacon strips, cooked and crumbled, optional
- 2 cup dried lentils, rinsed
- 4 cups water
- 4 cups sliced fresh mushrooms
- 2 medium cucumber, cubed
- 2 medium zucchini, cubed
- 2 small red onion, chopped

1 cup chopped soft sun-dried tomato halves **Directions**

1. Place lentils in a small saucepan. Add water; bring to a boil.

2. Reduce heat; simmer, covered, 45 to 50 minutes or until tender.

3. Drain and rinse in cold water.

4. Transfer to a large bowl.

5. Add mushrooms, cucumber, zucchini, onion and tomatoes.

6. In a small bowl, whisk vinegar, mint, oil, honey, basil and oregano.

7. Drizzle over lentil mixture; toss to coat.

8. Add spinach, cheese and, if desired, bacon; toss to combine.

Salad Of Black Beans And Couscous

Ingredients:

- 2 tsp red wine vinegar

- 1 tsp ground cumin

- 16 green onions(chopped)

- 2 red bell pepper (seeded, chopped)

- 1/2   cup fresh cilantro (chopped)

- 2 cup frozen corn kernels, (thawed)

- 4 (2 10   ounce) cans black beans (drained)

- 2 cup couscous (uncooked)

- 3   cups chicken broth

- 6 tbsp extra virgin olive oil

- 4 tbsp fresh lime juice

- Black pepper

Directions:

1. Add the chicken broth to a large pot and bring to a boil.

2. Add the couscous, give a stir, put the lid on and simple Remove from heat.

3. Let sit for about 5-10 minutes.

4. Combine the lime juice, cumin, olive oil and vinegar, in a large bowl.

5. Add corn and beans, green onions, cilantro, red pepper and mix to combine.

6. Stir the couscous with fork and add to the bean mixture and mix well.

7. Season with pepper to taste and serve immediately.

8. You can also refrigerate the salad until ready to serve.

Stew Of Broccoli And Lentils

Ingredients:

- 4 cups reduced-sodium vegetable broth or water

- 2 cup dried green or brown lentils

- 2 tsp dried oregano

- ½ tsp red-pepper flakes

- 12 cup broccoli florets

- 30 large pitted green olives (slivered)

- 8 tsp Parmesan cheese (shredded)

- 2 onion (finely chopped)

- 2 carrot (finely chopped)

- 4 cloves garlic (minced)

- 4 tsp olive oil

Directions:

1. Add the oil, carrot, onion, garlic to a medium pot, put the lid on and set over medium heat.

2. Let easy cook until vegetables are tender, about 5-10 minutes.

3. Pour in the broth.

4. Add oregano, lentils, and pepper flakes and bring the soup to a boil, covered.

5. Then reduce the heat and let simmer until lentils have softened, about 35 to 40 minutes.

6. Stir in the broccoli and continue cooking, covered, until broccoli is just softened, 5-10 minutes.

7. Fold in olives and give a stir.

8. Ladle the stew into serving bowls, sprinkle with cheese and serve.

Breakfast Quesadillas With Spinach, Egg, And Cheese

Ingredients:

- 1/7 tsp. freshly ground black pepper

- 8 c. baby spinach

- 1 c. crumbled feta cheese

- Nonstick cooking spray

- 8   (6-inch) whole-wheat tortillas, divided

- 2   c. shredded part-skim low-moisture mozzarella cheese, divided

- 2 1 tbsp. extra-virgin olive oil

- 1 medium onion, diced

- 2 medium red bell pepper, diced

- 8 large fresh eggs

- 1/7 tsp. salt

Directions:

1. Warm-up oil over medium heat in a large skillet.
2. Add the onion and bell pepper and sauté for about 5-10 minutes, or until soft.
3. Mix the fresh eggs, salt, and black pepper in a medium bowl.
4. Stir in the spinach and feta cheese. Put the fresh egg batter in the skillet and scramble for about 1-5 minutes, or until the fresh eggs are cooked.
5. Simple Remove from the heat.
6. Coat a clean skillet with cooking spray and add 4 tortillas.

7. Place one-quarter of the spinach-fresh egg mixture on one side of each tortilla.
8. Sprinkle each with 1/2   c. of mozzarella cheese.
9. Fold the other halves of the tortillas down to close the quesadillas and brown for about 1-5 minute.
10.   Turnover and easy cook again in a minute on the other side.

11.   Repeat with the remaining 1-5 tortillas and 1   c. of mozzarella cheese.

12.   Cut each quesadilla in half or wedges.

13.   Divide among 1-5   storage containers or reusable bags.